BECOMING THE QUEEN IN ME

A holistic guidebook to self-love & personal growth

By Haeley Mariah

MP | Experience

COPYRIGHT

ISBN: 9798589516364
Imprint: Independently published

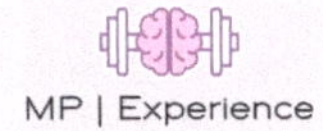

To all the women and girls out there who feel like they are mentally stuck in their ways. I empower you to free yourself.

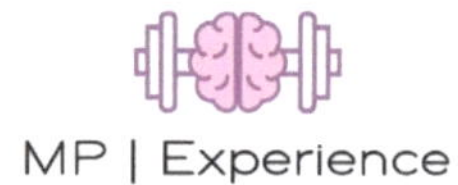

MP | Experience

Hello Queens!

I am super excited that you hold possession of this guidebook and all the gems that it has to offer. But I will be honest with you, none of the value in this guidebook will have an impact on your life until you are ready to receive this message fully. Wherever you are in your growth journey, this guidebook is here to ignite your path with blessings and support. If you think that you will read this guidebook and automatically your life will change, well, that ain't going to happen. Change happens overtime, but the **will** to change takes a second. That single choice to strive for a better tomorrow is what paves a brighter path. What will happen though, after reading this guidebook, is that a piece of your heart and soul will be touched, sparking hope into your future. Hope creates new beginnings through suffering. If you have been suffering in any way, shape or form then you are in the right place. I believe that everything happens for a reason. You are meant to be here now, reading and receiving all that this guidebook has to offer you. You manifested change, now your new beginning is here.

Don't worry! I got you, because I truly care about your holistic growth. If there are one or two things that I want you to take away from this guidebook, it is that YOU ARE STRONGER THAN YOU THINK and that YOU DESERVE TO BE TRULY HAPPY. No matter what anyone else thinks, never lose faith in the process of your growth.

Fellow Queens, I want you to hold your head high standing firmly on two feet while loving yourself unconditionally. You are destined for greatness and this world needs you at your best. So, let's progress into unapologetic self-confidence and self-love.

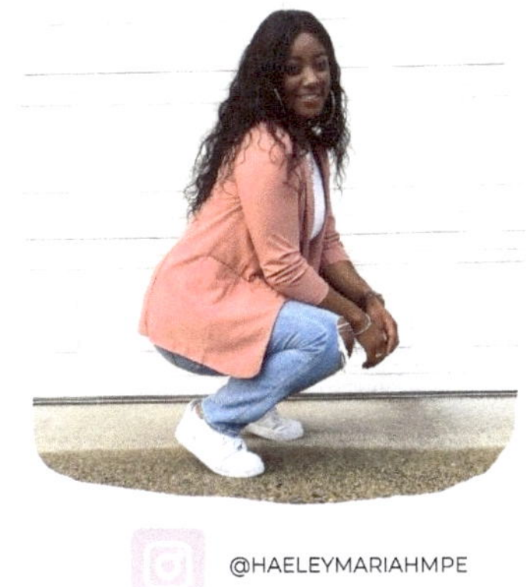

The journey to embracing your full Queen Powers flows from the alignment and harmony of your mind, body, soul and spirit. Keeping that in mind, The MPE uses a strong foundation of MINDSET, FITNESS AND NUTRITION to make that alignment possible and to create an enjoyable growth process that you will love and endure. In this guide, I will teach you and guide you through all of the tips and tricks I use to sustain a balanced, healthy and peaceful life.

You will learn healthier self-love habits that allow you to feel good, look good and regain self-control. Being kind, patient and loving are healthy habits that make us feel good!

The journey to self-love and personal growth is not smooth sailing but it is possible. It is the conscious choice to keep climbing your mountain every day.

Haeley Mariah xoxo

THE MP EXPERIENCE

IN ORDER TO BE YOUR BEST SELF YOU MUST FIRST FIND SELF-LOVE

There are no ifs, ands or buts about this one. Self-love is a right and a skill that must be obtained to sustain. As we just read, hope is creating new beginnings through suffering. We must walk through the valley before we can reach our mountain top, true for any success story. Queen's we have hope and vision. As much as we may not understand it yet, suffering is a natural part of life. We need suffering so we can feel and embrace comfort. A world without pain and suffering is an unrealistic fantasy world. There is no reality without pain and suffering. This falls under The Universal Law of Polarity - we cannot have up without down, good without bad, black without white, love without hate, and joy without suffering. This is duality. We have to know what we don't want to know what we do want, so we don't take the good for granted. There is no satisfying answer to the question of "why do good things happen to bad people?". All I know, experienced and have learned is that we truly desire comfort, the number one thing we need when we are suffering is comfort. So as you continue on your journey to self-love and personal growth keep pushing past the uncomfortable because something amazing is waiting for you on the other side pain.

Let's get back to hope. Hope is such a beautiful thing for the process it allows us to experience. Through suffering we endure, while we're enduring we are building character and through our new built character we are capable of creating our new beginnings with new insights. The most powerful aspect of hope is believing. Believing that new beginnings are possible, that a new lifestyle can be formed, new habits can be developed and a brighter future can be lived. Nothing new will come unless you truly BELIEVE that a new way of living and thinking is possible for you. According to the Cambridge Dictionary, self-efficacy is defined as "a person's belief that they can be successful when carrying out a particular task". While we are growing, learning new skills and stepping outside of our comfort zone, belief in our own potentiality (self-efficacy) is what makes this all possible for us. BELIEVE IN YOURSELF. If you struggle to believe in yourself, I want to remind you that we were created for greatness. What helps me believe is knowing and understanding that humans were created in the image of the higher power, the creator, God. God is love and his love is unfailing. Because we were made in his image this means that we are also love. But activating this love (power) is a choice, just how believing is a choice. Choose love over hate and always come from a place with love in your heart.

Introduction

Becoming The Queen In Me teaches you all about self-love and personal growth through three main health focus areas: mindset, fitness and nutrition. I want to help you regain a relationship with your mind, how you view your body and the food you consume.

Self-love is attainable and personal growth is sustainable. Let's grow together, inside and out, one day at a time.

CONTENTS

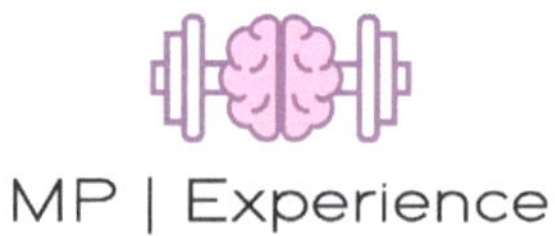

MP | Experience

CHAPTER 1
Behind the scenes

4 STEP PROCESS FOR
INTENTIONAL GROWTH

Healing through Self-Discovery

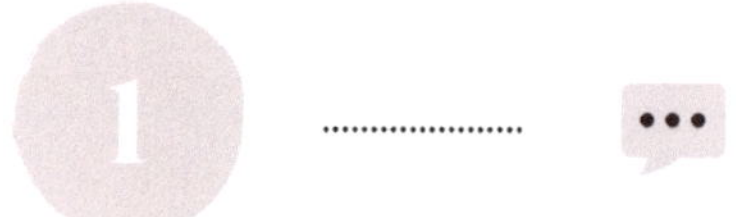

ACKNOWLEGDGE

Intentional growth starts by being brutally honest and aware of how we treat ourselves, the words we use to describe ourselves, what we're doing vs. not doing to heal ourselves, and recognizing the quality of our living and the trajectory of where our life is going. IT IS TIME TO WAKE UP from a negative way of living and thinking. Acknowledge where you are today so that you can watch yourself grow into the peaceful Queen you are meant to be.

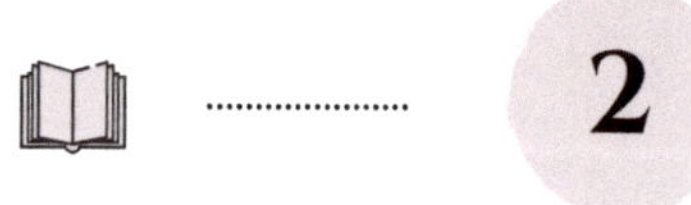

ACCEPT

REALITY CHECK! This is your one body, your one life, your one mind, and your one heart that you were blessed with. You cannot be anyone else and you will not be anyone else authentically. You are you! IT IS TIME TO ACCEPT ALL THAT YOU ARE. Once you can accept who you are for how you are then you can grow and flourish into your best self intentionally. Your best self WILL NOT come to light until you embrace who you naturally are. It is such a blessing that you are the only YOU in this world.

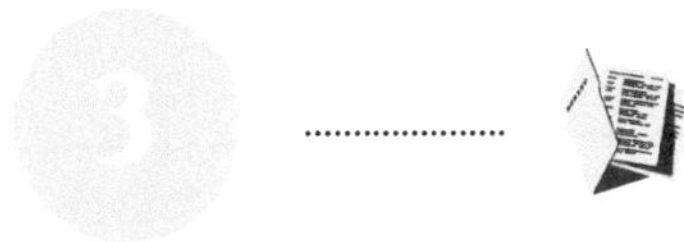

FORGIVE

We have to acknowledge and accept before we can forgive. This includes forgiving others AND ourselves. I am going to be honest with you. We will fall. Our feelings will get hurt and we will make mistakes. But we cannot continue to grow and rise UP until we forgive ourselves for what we did or did not do and to free our mind from the negative memories and the emotions attached to those negative memories. Forgiveness is freedom, personal freedom. Someone may hurt you and not even realize it, yet for all this time we are still holding on to the pain. This limits our growth. Forgive so you can move on and keep the memories without the negative feelings. Forgive yourself for handling life the best way you knew how in that moment. Forgive.

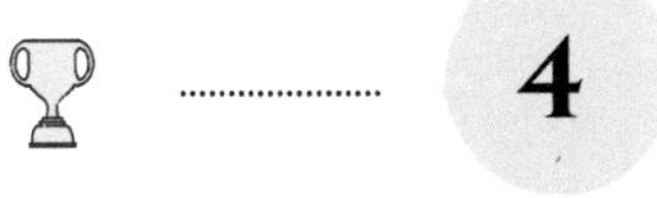

SELF-CULTIVATE

Never stop learning. NEVER. STOP. LEARNING. No seriously, never stop WANTING to learn. This is self-will. Finding the strength within yourself to DO, even if you might not want to, KNOWING that you WILL benefit greatly from that action. Do the things, surround yourself with the things, and cultivate the things that make you feel good. Never stop learning, discovering yourself, asking questions and exploring the true essence of who you are at your core. This is so important. When you stop WANTING TO LEARN then you are neglecting your right to develop your mind and capacities through your own efforts.

Authenticity is the daily practice of letting go of who we think we are supposed to be and embracing who we truly are.
-Brene Brown

3 GROWTH TIPS
for a Growing Queen

TIP #1

CREATE DAILY ROUTINES

Let's keep things simple. Daily routines are a set of actions that we repeat daily. We know what to do and when to do it. There is immense simplicity in daily routines. I want to help you simplify your life with healthy routines that will help set the vibe and tone for each day and each night. We do this through morning and night routines. These routines don't have to be too crazy or too time consuming but are things you truly believe you are capable of doing each day, knowing that they will bring you peace, joy and happiness. The idea here is to feel good and grow intentionally, correct? So, help yourself keep things simple. Spend some quality time alone creating your unique routine, adding things that will help your mind rest and be stress free. Make each routine make sense in your own life. My best advice here: add actions that promote self-love in both your morning and your night routines. When we act in love, we are not hating and hate weighs heavy on our hearts. Our goal is to be prepared and not perfect. There is no shame if some days we miss out on our routine or choose to do something else. THE INTENT FOR SETTING A POSITIVE TONE IS THE REAL GAME CHANGER.

MORNING ROUTINE EXAMPLES:
- Set your alarm a few minutes earlier to incorporate some sort of morning meditation or prayer
- Manifest some love towards different (or the same) people every morning
- Drink a herbal tea to start the day
- Listen to your favorite inspirational song or podcast
- Read your favorite inspirational quote
- Read the Bible

NIGHT ROUTINE EXAMPLES:
- Creative visualization (meditate)
- Read 15 minutes
- Drink a calming tea ex. Chamomile
- Take a bath or shower while listening to calming music

TIP #2

FIND YOUR WHY

There is no pressure and no timeline on your growth. Come into your self-discovery at your own pace. A helpful tip: once you have acknowledged that you are ready to start making an intentional effort towards your growth, I recommend thinking about and finding your WHY. Let your WHY be your underlying layer for the days you want to give up, the days and times that life feels too hard, and to help give yourself clarity in decision making. Let your WHY ground you and refocus you on what truly matters to you at your core. Spending the time to really think about and understand your underlying WHY that drives you is really important. Why do you want to grow and make healthier changes? Why now? What's different? My best advice here: start by reflecting on what puts a smile on your face, makes you want to get up out of bed every morning and be your best self. What drives you internally and externally to actually get you up and to make royal moves? Your WHY can forever evolve just like you, forever evolving.

SOME EXAMPLES:
- My WHY: "so I can use my experiences to help uplift the experiences of those around me"
- ex. Internal motivations: you want to be become your best self, you want to feel better, you want to love yourself unconditionally, to feel comfortable in your own skin, you are ready to put your mind at ease
- ex. External motivations: your family and those who love you, you want to be a role model for your children or siblings, you want to be a better wife, girlfriend or friend. Your business reflects you well-being.

TIP #3

NEVER STOP LEARNING

Plant your seed and water it with knowledge. Knowledge is the most powerful force a human being can obtain. Knowledge is a force that is something to be reckoned with and is used to change your life for the better or the worse. Finding your own knowledge is finding your own truths. Knowledge is our shape shifter. Feed your mind with truths that help you become, evolve, adapt, transform and change. We cannot become something we do not know we want to become. Knowledge gives us this direction, opening that door to endless possibilities. Knowledge gives us hope, freedom of choice, self-control and a sense of who we are. What are you choosing to do with your time? Time is a valuable thing that you can spend but cannot buy. Are you trying to distract yourself from being and feeling in the present moment? Running away from all of your possibilities and dreams? Remember, I am choosing to call you out to help you grow, not to make you feel worse about yourself. If you are currently feeling attacked by these words then maybe that is a good thing. My best advice: swallow your pride, take this knowledge in for what it is, and regain power over your life. Queen, I want to see you thrive! We must get uncomfortable to get comfortable in a better place. Never stop wanting to learn.

SOME GUIDANCE:
- Join my Personal Growth Program
- Read personal development/ self help books
- Listening to motivating and encouraging podcasts
- Watch Videos to better understand topics or concepts
- EDUCATE YOURSELF WITH THINGS THAT ADD VALUE TO YOUR GROWTH RATHER THAN DISTRACT YOU FROM ACTUALLY HEALING
- Don't waste your time on things that hinder or deter your self-love and personal growth
  - ex. aimlessly scrolling social media

CHAPTER 2
Set your foundations

BE OPEN, HONEST
And Raw

If we are going to create any significance and life long changes in our lives then we have to be open to hearing new insights.

I fell in love with this quote written by an Ancient Mystic "the only thing that burns in Hell is self-will". When I first heard this quote in The Kingdom is Yours: Healing Tears Podcast by Joshua Luke Smith I was stopped in confusion. I had to listen to this quote over and over again until it sunk deep into my soul and spirit. Well, when I broke it down, Hell is the opposite of Heaven; the highest, holiest, graceful and peaceful place that God created. I have learned that God is love, and love resides in all of us, activated upon conscious choice and will. So it only made sense that if God is love, then God resides in all us. And if God made Heaven through love, then Hell must have been created through hate and fear, the opposites of love. Based on my understanding of Heaven, Hell meant to me, the lowest, fear driven, and self-limiting place that holds us captive of our sins. Wow, that was a lot of words but I don't apologize for it. The point I am trying to get across is that the lack of self-will is essentially the lack of truly living. The lack of self-will is the only thing that prevents us from fully experiencing the goodness available to us, almost like living in hell. If we are not living in peace then my understanding is that we are living in fear and fear is Hell driven.

After proficient reflecting and analyzing of the experiences from my own life and the lives of all of my clients, I have come to the conclusion that the lack of self-will is fear driven. We procrastinate, self-sabotage and create limiting beliefs of ourselves and world due to fear. If we continue to let fear be the reason we are not wanting to make uplifting and life changing changes then we are consciously choosing to live in mental Hell.

I am here to share words with you that you may not want to hear but need to hear to shed light on the truths of your heart and soul. We, our thoughts, our beliefs, our actions, behaviours and attitudes, are the only things that is stopping us from living in peace; our best, most authentic and most successful versions of ourselves. Fear is an illusion and you can change your narrative.

Live fully, trust your process and be fearless.

DAILY RITUALS
It's the effort that counts

The simplest and most effective way that I have learned to sustain my self-love and personal growth journey is through daily rituals. To really break it down, daily rituals are just intentional actions, behaviors and thoughts that you practice daily. How I describe it: daily rituals are healthy habits that, when done consistently, allow your body to feel inner peace from doing things that make you feel good. It's how you perceive your actions. Are they mundane chores that just need to be completed, or are they actions that bring meaning, learning or joy into your life? It's all about your mindset.

EVERY MORNING JUST ASK YOURSELF
"DO YOU WANT TO BE HAPPY?

Is happiness deserved, or do we have to earn it? I say that happiness is deserved, but we have to want to have it. We have to want to do the things that actually help us feel true happiness and inner peace - healthy habits - such as being kind to ourselves through empowering self-talk, moving our body daily so our body can move for us, nourishing our mind and body with food that will add value not take value, reflecting on our actions and thoughts so we can be aware of them, and of course, giving ourselves the space and freedom to feel peace every day, making this feeling mandatory. _If we want to feel good, then it is our responsibility to do the work to make sure that we feel good. You have to want to do the work. This is the only natural way._

These are the daily rituals that I practice and teach:
- Daily Positive Affirmations
  - self-talk
- Daily Body Movement
  - fitness
- Daily Mindful Eating
  - nutrition
- Daily Self-Reflection
  - mindset
- Daily Mandatory Period of Peace
  - breath work

Go to www.haeleymariahmpe.com to fill out your 1:1 online 12 Week Personal Growth Program application form. Also, check the website to join my next 21 Day Healthy Habits Challenge where we learn and practice these daily rituals together.

WE HAVE THE
Right & Responsibility

We all have the right and responsibility to live the life we truly desire. We have the right and responsibility to self-love and personal growth. We have the right and responsibility to positive thoughts, faith, and self-belief. We have the right and responsibility to take intentional action of the things we have control over and how we respond versus react to certain situations. We have the right and responsibility to love, happiness and inner peace. I understand that not everyone has the same privilege, access to books, healthier nutritional options or even a healthy environment to live in. But this does not take away our responsibility of showing up as our best selves everyday in whatever matter that means to each individual. This does not give us the right to stop trying or caring for a better tomorrow, remember tomorrow is not promised. Anything is possible if you are willing to make it possible for yourself. We have the right to life and the responsibility to live fully. Take every roadblock and hurdle as a challenge. A common quote that my clients will hear me say is "seek challenge to get change". As we learned in The Intentional Growth Step number 2, is it not our right to be comparing ourselves to anyone else, or anyone else's living situation. All of our roadblocks and hurdles may look different, but it is a fact that we all have them. Do YOUR best to live YOUR best life by first WANTING to do what it takes to BE your best self.

It may be hard to hear, but it is YOUR responsibility to break through excuses and make whatever needs to happen happen. Remember, this is your only life. Do the best you can with what you have. Make the healthier choices where you can, be kind to yourself when you can, and move your body when you can. It is YOUR job to create happiness and peace, to find your light in the darkness. It is YOUR job to focus on your thoughts, to care about your thoughts and to change your thoughts when need be. It is YOUR job to get up, even if you don't want to and do whatever it is you need to get done for the day. It is YOUR job to stop procrastinating. Queen, if you are sitting around waiting for someone else to do what you won't do, you will forever be waiting in Hell.

You are the direct reflection of your efforts... were you aware of this? I really don't doubt for a second that you didn't. I believe that we all have all of the answers that we need inside of us, we just have to be willing to do the work to find those answers and then make the effort to apply those answers. This is self-will.

Your intentional efforts are the key to your success and holding yourself responsible for your actions is what changes your lifestyle. The knowing is one thing, but the doing... oh honey, trust! I get it, I feel like this is why we beat ourselves up so often. We know what we need to be doing, what makes us feel good and what doesn't, yet we do or don't do it anyways. Sometimes right away, but not always, we feel guilty, then we hold onto that guilt to the point where we stop trusting ourselves. Dang, I know, I am calling you out but I don't apologize for that. I want you to know, and realize, so you can grow.

Every person that comes into your life is meant to show and teach you something new about yourself. Believe it or not, the relationships that you keep are a reflection of the relationship you have with yourselves. So if you are stuck in any toxic relationships (family, friendships, significant others , or food) I advice you start focusing on how you treat yourself. Show other people the only love you are willing to receive by first showing yourself the only love you are willing to give yourself. Healthy relationships start and end with self-love. It is hard to create healthy habits but it something that we all must do to sustain inner peace, joy and happiness. There are no other natural options that won't steal your peace.

SELF-LOVE IS NOT...

- numbing or avoiding your feelings
- staying in toxic relationships by refusing to walk away
- comparing yourself to others in a negative way
- talking down on yourself or negatively labelling yourself
- stress eating
- giving up
- weighing yourself everyday
- procrastinating
- a sedentary lifestyle
- physically hurting yourself
- starving yourself
- refusing to read, gain knowledge or ask questions
- choosing not to care
- sleeping with men or women to feel better about yourself
- staying in a career you hate
- having children to find purpose
- something you have to do alone

Loving yourself and rebuilding a relationship with yourself is not an easy thing. Do not feel like you have to go on this journey alone.

CHAPTER 3
Now What?

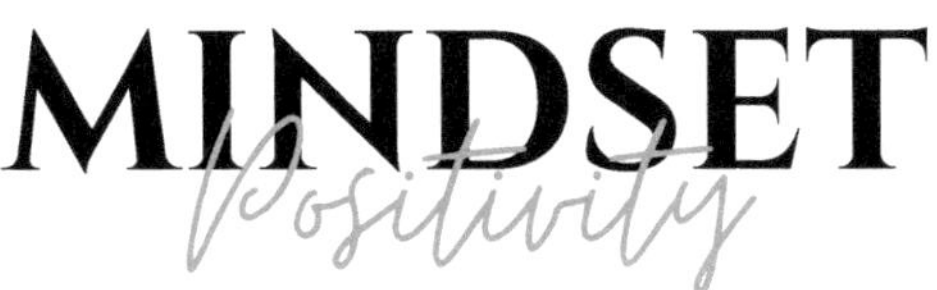

Mindset is everything. I am sure you have heard that before, but do you believe in it? Do you believe that your current reality is the byproduct of your thoughts? Do you believe that what you constantly think, the words you continuously say to and about yourself, shapes your today? Do you believe that when you think of bad things or when bad things happen to you, when you feel down about yourself and your very existence, that this is all a result of your past thinking? Are these just coincidences to you or do you see that everything happens for a reason? I will be honest with you. I used to believe in luck, that some people had it and some never would. That there was no purpose to anything and that things just kind of randomly happened. Some people drew the happy and peaceful straws while others drew the unhappy and depressed straws. I thought the toxic way I was thinking and living was just how my life was meant to be lived. Boy, was I ever wrong! Nothing changed for me until I changed my mind from a fixed mindset to a growth mindset; from understanding that anything can come from nothing. I chose to recreate my narrative and you can do the same thing too.

I learned that every word that comes out of my mouth, and every thought that I think, holds immense power and shapes the success of my future. "For as [s]he thinks in [her] heart, so is [s]he" (Proverbs 23:7). This is one of my favourite bible verses that I will forever repeat to myself. We are what we think we are, and we feel how we think about feeling. Having a positive mindset is a choice, a very daunting choice but a very worthwhile and freeing choice, one that needs to be made every day as every day is a new beginning. Think of your thoughts and thinking as mental powers. Every word we say, or think, holds energy, positive or negative. Positive energy holds uplifting and empowering weight while negative energy holds stressful, limiting and discouraging weight. Stress will slowly kill you, literally so DO NOT GIVE YOUR POWER AWAY. Do not give anyone else the power to effect your emotions or energy. If you know who you are then no one else can tell you who you are or knock you off the course of your newly paved path. How you think of yourself is like a force field that no one else should be able to break. We are Queens right? So guard yourself at all times with your own view of self. This is why being on a journey to self-love and personal growth is extremely important. You are taking the steps to build your owners manual so you know exactly who you are inside and out, loving all of you for who you are unconditionally.

BE THE BEST
Of Your Emotions

This leads us into our emotions. If you want to feel good please, feel good. Please free yourself from your own Mental Well that is holding your peace captive. If someone or something tries to come for your peace, breath first so you can respond rather than react. When we react we are not in control, when we respond we have taken the time to process before we make our next move. Remember, we can only control ourselves and nothing else. Most of us struggle with this because we like to have control over the things we have no actual control over, such as other people and outcomes, relatable but unrealistic. My advice, don't waste your energy. Redirect that energy on upholding positive thoughts. Carry love in your heart to cast out all fears of the unknown. When we act in love there is no room for fear or hate.

Oh ya! Another big lesson that I learned, don't avoid or run from your emotions. Jeez, this is a big one. If you don't deal with your emotions now, I promise they will resurface when you least expect it. There is no shame or guilt in feeling things fully, so please do yourself justice and feel all that you need to feel when you need to feel them. Feel and acknowledge, step 1 of our Intentional Growth Steps. Live free of shame for shame is a soul sucking emotion.

I have also learned that as we think positively or negatively that our brain literally changes shapes. Each new thought paves a new path in our brain. When we think a positive thought this tends to lead to another positive thought and hopefully another. When we think a negative thought this also tends to lead to another negative thought. I believe that this is how we get stuck and trapped by our own mental limitations in our Mental Well—from a downward spiral of continuous negative thoughts. Free your mind one positive and empowering thought at a time. Catch yourself slipping with positive affirmations. When you notice yourself thinking or saying something negative about yourself replace that thought with a positive thought to stay on a positive path. Life is about picking yourself up every time you fall, and not expecting someone else to do it for you. We are not meant to stay at the bottom of our Mental Well. I believe we are meant to be at the peak of our potentials. Become your highest conscious self by being your most resilient and present self. Mindset is everything. This ain't no joke. Having a growth mindset is a form of self-love.

FITNESS
Body Movement

Body movement is like my therapy, as if it is the medicine that rebalances my well-being. The number one value that I have learned from exercising is to be fully present in everything that you do. Essentially this just means to fully be where you are today. If you cannot be present where you are today why do you think you will be present as a stronger version of yourself? Start today, learn the skills today and take this journey one day at a time. Being present where you are today births new beginnings else where. It is easy to get discouraged while working out from not seeing results at the rate that we desire, but hang in there and have hope. Live a life that will cost you who you are today.

I use fitness as a tool to increase my mind-body connection and to stabilize my emotions. Is having good health something that is important to you? And be honest with yourself. For many of us the answer will be no and that is your current truth. But I will say one thing, a sedentary (inactive) lifestyle is an unhappy lifestyle. I want you to be happy and to live your BEST life not a mediocre life. I believe that everyone is deserving of living their best life. Intentionally move your body daily to activate your four happy chemicals: serotonin, dopamine, oxytocin and endorphin. These are natural chemicals in the brain that impact our happiness. If being happy and at peace is your goal, which I highly recommend that it is, then I encourage you to mindfully move your body daily.

This intention helps you manage stress, anxiety and depression, improves your quality of sleep and aids in weight management, along with many other health benefits. Most of us are looking for the light at the end of the tunnel. What you must realize is that road blocks will come and test your ability to be strong and endure to the end. We need them. Finding the strength to overcome these obstacles starts with mindful thinking. Take your thoughts to a mindful place where positivity and encouragement allow you to propel your body and your life past the temptations that exist. Growth comes from making hard decisions for the sake of your future. One of the aspects that I did not tap into yet because I wanted your full focus was the "4 Pillars of Health". These pillars are important to me because through their alignment and harmony I was able to find my moral compass. When I began this journey as a Fitness Trainer, Life Coach and Nutrition Coach, it was tough to build a foundation I could stand on as a woman. I had to search within myself and find answers that would allow me to be at peace with myself first. When I found peace for myself, I was able to impact thousands of lives by using these pillars to build structure.

MIND-BODY-SOUL-SPIRIT

These pillars of health are resourceful concepts that focus on holistic growth, strengthening your mind and your body through the alignment of your mind, body, soul and spirit. I've practiced these mindfulness tips over the last decade in preparation for this guidebook. I've found these pillars to be the building blocks of my growth journey and I want to help you facilitate your own journey. In a sedentary lifestyle, you will find yourself inside a lot, probably laying down or sitting and probably on your phone, computer or watching tv. No matter where you are in your house or apartment, I want you to focus on creating helpful reminders for yourself to move daily and keep a level mind. I am a huge fan of sticky notes on my walls. This is another step in the right direction. Next, find your strength to exercise even when you don't want to. Your body movement is crucial for your growth and well-being. I have attached a 30-day body movement challenge. These exercises can be done at home, or in the gym, with or without weights. If you choose to partake in this challenge, set the right intention and make a commitment to yourself, that everyday you will at least try! 10% effort is more than 0% effort.

There are 24 hours in a day. That momentary workout will allow your body to elevate in health and wealth and your mind to a euphoric high. Most times we forget about how strong our bodies are when we begin physical activity. You will only be as strong as your mind wants you to be. So, remove all the bad thoughts and excuses from your mind as we enter the beginning stages of your growth journey or continue from the work you have already put in.

I do not coach fitness for the sole purpose of helping people lose weight, I coach people to help them live in peace and to love themselves unconditionally. Body positivity is the real deal. It is way too easy to scroll on Instagram or TikTok and compare yourself and your life to everyone that you see. "Wow she's beautiful, I wish I looked like____, I wish I was as happy as____". Remember point number two of our Intentional Growth Steps? Acceptance. THIS IS YOUR ONE BODY AND LIFE so treat your palace with respect. Move your body with respect and nourish your body with respect. If you want to feel comfortable and confident in the skin you're in, while losing or gaining a few pounds, then a holistic approach and your intentions are what you need to really focus on.

Body movement looks different for different people so find what works for you and what makes you feel happy and accomplished. If you are going to do a workout, be fully present. If you are going for a walk, a run, or a bike ride, be fully present. If you are at a sports practice, in a spin, dance or yoga class then be fully present. If you are stretching, yup you guessed it, be fully present. Queen, if you are simply walking to the kitchen to make a healthy meal and you notice you haven't moved all day then you better strut yourself to that kitchen with the intent of "this is my 10% for the day, and I am going to enjoy all 10% of it" you can even throw in a little dance while you're at it.

Just move intently. Why I teach the 10% body movement rule is so that you can hold yourself accountable for your actions in hopes that, on some days, that 10% leads to 20%, 50% or higher. If you strive for a 10% minimum of body movement daily then you are not only thriving but also developing and applying healthy habits that aid in increasing your personal growth in daily increments. I recommend starting with 2-3 scheduled workouts a week with a minimum of 10% movement on the other days. Staying active, healthy and fit are forms of self-love.

> *Today, do what others won't so tomorrow you can accomplish what others can't.*
> -Simone Biles, Gymnast

30-DAY FITNESS CHALLENGE

Your results are a direct reflection of your effort. YOU GOT THIS!!

1.
10 Squats
10 Jumping Jacks
10 Heel Touches

2.
20 Squats
20 Jumping Jacks
20 Heel Touches

3.
30 Squats
30 Jumping Jacks
30 Heel Touches

4.
40 Squats
40 Jumping Jacks
40 Heel Touches

5.
50 Squats
50 Jumping Jacks
50 Heel Touches

6.
10 Alt. Lunges
10 Leg Lifts
10 Crunches

7.
20 Alt. Lunges
20 Leg Lifts
20 Crunches

8.
30 Alt. Lunges
30 Leg Lifts
30 Crunches

9.
40 Alt. Lunges
40 Leg Lifts
40 Crunches

10.
50 Alt. Lunges
50 Leg Lifts
50 Crunches

11.
10 Russian Twists
10 Push Ups
10 Sumo Squats

12.
20 Russian Twists
20 Push Ups
20 Sumo Squats

13.
30 Russian Twists
30 Push Ups
30 Sumo Squats

14.
40 Russian Twists
40 Push Ups
40 Sumo Squats

15.
50 Russian Twists
50 Push Ups
50 Sumo Squats

16.
10 sec Plank
10 Side Lunge
10 Tricep Dip

17.
20 sec Plank
20 Side Lunge
20 Tricep Dip

18.
30 sec Plank
30 Side Lunge
30 Tricep Dip

19.
40 sec Plank
40 Side Lunge
40 Tricep Dip

20.
50 Plank
50 Side Lunge
50 Tricep Dip

21.
10 Two Feet Side Hops
10 Tent Push up
10 Reverse Crunch

22.
20 Two Feet Side Hops
20 Tent Push up
20 Reverse Crunch

23.
30 Two Feet Side Hops
30 Tent Push up
30 Reverse Crunch

24.
40 Two Feet Side Hops
40 Tent Push up
40 Reverse Crunch

25.
50 Two Feet Side Hops
50 Tent Push up
50 Reverse Crunch

26.
10 Glute Bridge
10 Bird Dog
10 High Plank Jack

27.
20 Glute Bridge
20 Bird Dog
20 High Plank Jack

28.
30 Glute Bridge
30 Bird Dog
30 High Plank Jack

29.
40 Glute Bridge
40 Bird Dog
40 High Plank Jack

30.
50 Glute Bridge
50 Bird Dog
50 High Plank Jack

Join **The MPE Monthly Membership** for exercise video library, motivational text messages, emails, a FB community support group, unlimited motivational boot camps, boot camp recordings, first access and discount to more guidebooks and challenges.

www.haeleymariahmpe.com

NUTRITION
Mindful Eating

First things first: eating healthy is a form of self-respect. Respect your mind and your body by feeding it with good energy.

FOOD IS ENERGY. PROTECT YOUR ENERGY BY EATING MINDFULLY.

Weight is not my main focus BUT to really break things down: weight loss = consuming less energy than we use, weight gain = consuming more energy than we use. Basically, what and how much we eat in a day has a certain effect on the growth of our physical body and the healing of our mental well-being. So, start by knowing what YOUR personal goals are and act accordingly. EAT TO FUEL YOUR INTERNAL POWERS. When it comes to losing weight or gaining weight, I always start by asking my clients WHY. Remember Growth Tip number two that we learned? Knowing WHY you want something gives you power, clarity and authenticity in your choices. You are doing X Y Z because YOU want to and not because you feel you have too. I know that for many of us our nutrition and food choices are some of our biggest weaknesses. It's hard and has the potential to cause stress so we give in to what's easy, junk. The best nutritional advice that I can give you is: EAT WHEN YOU ARE HUNGRY and EAT FOR NEED. North Americans as a whole consume waaayy more food than our bodies are meant to sustain. On the opposite side, we tend to restrict ourselves from eating as a form of punishment when we are struggling to love ourselves. Eating healthy is a form of self-love.

The purpose of this section of the guide is to help you reduce some of that stress around eating and to rebuild a healthy relationship with the food you eat and, of course, with yourself. I personally do not coach diets or support diet culture. I coach mindful, intuitive eating with self-will and self-discipline components. Why? Because every body is different with different needs. There is not one set in stone eating regime that will work for everyone, so trial and error is huge. I find that this is a less stress, less anxious and less emotional way of eating and living. I believe that this style of eating allows us to regain control over our actions, to fight off temptations and to feel confident in our choices.

REBUILD YOUR RELATIONSHIP
With Food

So now you're probably wondering "okay cool, now what?". Well, to really simplify things each meal should aim to have protein, vegetables, carbs and healthy fats. This helps us create a solid energy balance. Yes, I said vegetables. Many of us may struggle finding the love for eating vegetables, you are not alone. But I want to remind you that our ultimate goal here is self-love and personal growth. Correct me if I am wrong, when we eat junk we feel like junk? And when we eat clean we feel clean? I will gladly take the role of calling you out yet again. As much as you may not like eating healthy, in order to achieve the health goals, self-love goals, and personal growth goals that you desire YOU MUST eat healthy. You MUST break that stubbornness of "It doesn't taste good so I don't want too" or "I am too lazy to cook so I will eat out". Okay fair, but those just sound like excuses to me. Again correct me if I am wrong.

 As we know, the journey to self-love and personal growth IS NOT EASY. Please don't think that it is supposed to be easy or that if things get hard that you should quit. This is where self-will and self-discipline come into play. Again, we are not striving for perfection, only intentional effort, so do not forget that balance is necessary. Eat what you like consciously. Know what you are eating and why so there is no room to beat yourself up afterwards. OWN YOUR CHOICES. LEARN FROM YOUR CHOICES and make changes as you need. So yes, if you want the cookie then eat the cookie. But if we are eating cookies every day and gaining weight, don't you dare try to point your fingers at anyone else. You knew what you were doing while eating all those cookies. Breath, it's okay, make your next choice a healthy choice. To break down mindful eating... really look at the words. MINDFUL EATING... The idea here is to mindfully think and create dialogue around what we are putting into our body. Awareness. I encourage you to think in terms of "we are what we eat" because there is so much truth in this quote. It's a bit cliché, but it is true! Build your owner's manual around what food makes you feel good and what foods don't. You be the judge of what is best for your body. Mindful eating is a form of self-love.

TRY THESE
Tips & Tricks

- Eat slowly and mindfully
- Drink some water before eating
- Ask yourself if you are hungry or bored?
- Ask yourself if you are hungry or stressed?
- On a scale of 1-10 how hungry am I?
- Physical hunger and fullness checks
- Did you just eat?
- Does your stomach hurt?
- Eat to 80% full
- Don't eat until you are stuffed
- Eating slowly is CRUCIAL
- When you are out and start to stress, think "MAKE IT HOME before eating" then have whatever you want to eat when you're home
- this eliminates stress Fast Food eating
- OR keep healthy snacks in the car, I love me some good car snacks
- Eliminate impulse junk eating and the emotions attached
- Give love to your food while cooking. As we know, energy matters. Cook and prep your food with good energy so you feel it while consuming.
- Bless your food while eating
- Always have a water bottle with you, this will help you actually drink the water and can be used to test if you are actually hungry or just thirsty.
- Self dialogue before eating
- Ask yourself if you are really hungry and why
- Allow yourself to have treats, there is nothing wring with treats in reasonable moderations. Eat the cookie girl, just be mindful of what the cookie is doing in your body. No shame no guilt, just enjoy and eat it in peace.
- The goal is to make conscious choices when eating to remove any impulse, guilt or shame after the fact.
- Fruits are best in the morning/ day through smoothie or eating the fruit alone (this doesn't mean that you can't eat fruit at night, because you can)
- Salads and smoothies are great light breakfast/brunch/lunch options

POWER SWEET SALAD

It's Healthy & It Tastes Good

INGREDIENTS

VEGGIES:

Chopped Lettuce
Baby Kale
Arugula
Radish Slices
Shaved Carrots
Shopped Bell Peppers
Chopped Tomatoes

TOPPINGS:

Roasted Walnuts
Roasted Pecans
Roasted Pistachios
Roasted Sunflower seeds
Roasted Pumpkin seeds
Hemp seeds
Chopped figs
Chopped dates

DRESSING:

Half of avocado
Avocado oil
Agave Syrup
Key lime or lemon

DIRECTIONS

Prep the veggies then place in eating bowl, sprinkle hemp seeds. In a small frying pan use extra virgin olive oil and add the "roasted toppings" with a drizzle of agave syrup. Stir for 5 minutes. In a small bowl mix half of an avocado, avocado oil to preferred dressing consistency, drizzle balsamic vinegar, drizzle agave syrup, squeeze half of key like or lemon. Mix all ingredients together & enjoy!

GOAL SETTING
With Intention

5 Step Method To Attain Your Goals:
from the Monk Who Sold His Ferrari

1. FORM A CLEAR MENTAL PICTURE OF YOUR OUTCOME

This can be done through mediation, creative visualization, prayer

2. CREATE A LITTLE PRESSURE BEHIND IT

Tell someone your plan, let them laugh at you. Make your outcome a MUST despite what anyone else thinks. If you truly believe in this goal then that is all that matters. MAKE IT HAPPEN.

3. SET A DEADLINE, COMMIT IT TO PAPER

There is magic when you bring pen to paper, old fashioned style. Write it out.

4. THE MAGIC RULE OF 21!

- *It takes 21 days to create a habit.*
- *No pressure, take it one day at a time.*
- *Tracking your progress creates visual growth which helps you persevere*

5. ENJOY THE DAILY PROCESS

We long so deeply to be the best version of ourselves and have that end goal. But, really appreciate each day for THIS, the everyday grind, is where the magic happens. Let go of the stress and be present. You got this, we all got this!

WRITE YOUR GOALS:

<u>In your own notebook,</u> answer these in terms of "what I need and want to be the best version of myself". What does that look like? Paint a mental picture with these goals. After writing down your goals, manifest them through meditation, creative visualization, or prayer. ATUALLY DO THIS! Do it right now so you don't forget.

1. <u>Emotional Goals</u>- ex. no negativity, stress will not enter my body, I am calm and confident in all situations, I am aware when my emotions change and can block it out if negative

2. <u>Materialistic Goals</u>- ex. what are some musts in your dream home? do you have a dream car? things you've always wanted if money was no issue. Dream career or business?

3. <u>Physical Goals</u>- ex. how do you want to feel physically? what about your health? Does anything physically need to heal?

4. <u>Spiritual Goals</u>- ex. how do you want to feel spiritually? what are your spiritual beliefs? what ways do you want to grow spiritually? What energy do you want to invite into your life? do you want to be spiritually connected?

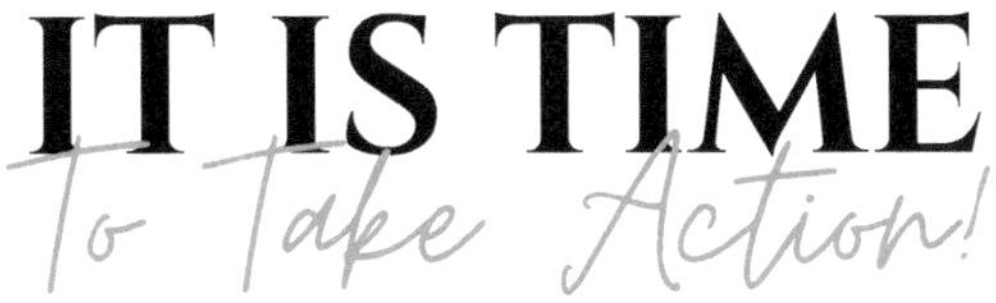

GET UNCOOMFORTABLE TO GET COMFORTABLE IN A BETTER PLACE.

So. You have made it this far, now what? Is this when you close the book, put it away and forget all of the knowledge and insight obtained? I sure hope not. If you are serious about your journey to self-love and personal growth then now is when we start to actually do something about it.

Here is what you have:
- your 30 day fitness challenge
- a power sweet salad to try - let me know how you like it!
- your goals to write in your notebook
- The MPE Membership to join so you can stay active and engaged in an accountability and support group where you can ask your questions, share your wins, stay present, and attend/watch lives, guest speaker talks and informational videos
  - membership includes:
    - motivational texts and emails
    - FB accountability and support group
    - unlimited boot camp access
    - boot camp recordings
    - exercise video library
    - first access and discount pricing for more books and live challenges
- A 12 week 1:1 Personal Growth Program to join
- A website to visit - www.haeleymariahmpe.com
- 2 Instagram pages to follow, engage with and be influenced by
  - @haeleymariahmpe
  - @showlove.official
- this guidebook to reference back to whenever you need it

QUEEN! YOU. HAVE. OPTIONS.
NO EXCUSES. *GO OFF!*

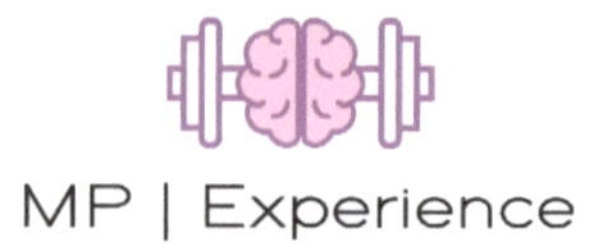

WHAT THE HECK DOES THE MPE STAND FOR?

The MPE stands for "The Mental and Physical Experience". This is a holistic experience that is set in place to provide women and girls with a wide variety of ways to gain or rebuild their internal powers; the God in them.

The MPE wants to see you be your very best self. The MPE believes that an increase in self-love and personal growth will in return make the world a better and brighter place, one person at a time.

The MPE will help you reshape your view of self, teach you healthy daily habits and how to show other people how to treat you best, and creates a positive, uplifting and supportive community for like-minded Queens like yourself.

The MPE is your journey to self-love and personal growth.

Don't forget to join the MPE membership and FB group.

www.haeleymariahmpe.com

*Join **The MPE Monthly Membership** for motivational text messages, emails, FB community support group, unlimited motivational boot camps, exercise video library, boot camp recordings, first access and discount to more guidebooks and challenges.*

ABOUT THE AUTHOR

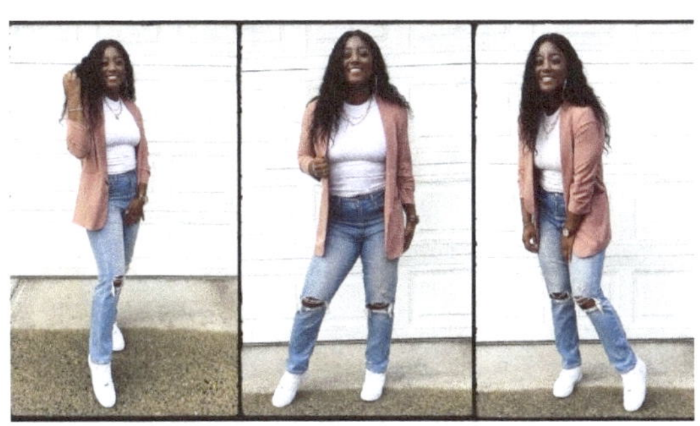

For over 10 years I have been working closely with youth, both girls and boys, as a Sports Coach, Mentor, Team Leader, Residential Youth Care Worker and Youth Counsellor. For about 8 years now I have been actively studying and learning about humanities, why people do what they do, personal growth and the human experience as a whole. Today, I am a Mentor, Fitness Trainer, Mindset Coach, Life Coach and Nutrition Coach working closely with women and girls. I founded The MP Coaching Experience back in 2018 with my first 1:1 client and The MPE has been growing rapidly ever since. I consider myself a visionary. I have always had this unique ability to see potential and the trajectory of those around me. While battling my own experiences in my past with being diagnosed with Severe Depression, I am blessed to say that I have found unconditional inner peace and self-love in my own personal growth journey. I use the knowledge obtained from my BA in Criminology and background in Counselling Psychology, my certifications, my life experiences and my relationship with God to create a holistic growth experience in the form of guidebooks, challenges, pop-up boot camps and my 12-week personal growth program which are all unique and effective and designed to help women and girls feel good, look good and regain self-control.

I move with faith and spirituality for a holistic growth experience empowering women and girls to uncover their fullest potentiality as they journey towards becoming their most authentic selves. This is what makes me stand out. I am proficient in creating an enjoyable holistic growth experience that you will love and admire, creating sustainable inner peace and self-awareness. My focus is to increase your mental and physical strength so that you can become the best and most successful version for yourself. Let's break barriers and grow together, inside and out. One day at a time!

Have questions?

Send me an email!
haeleymariah.mpe@gmail.com
www.haeleymariahmpe.com

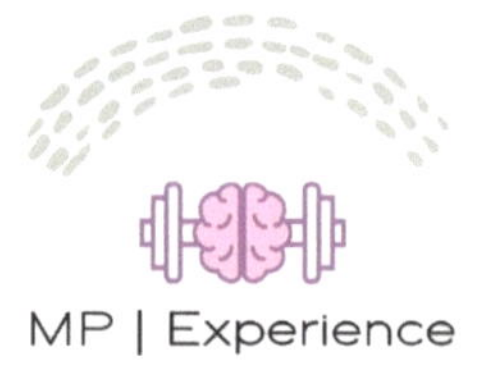

CHANGE THE WAY YOU THINK TO CHANGE THE WAY YOU LIVE.

WE ARE *QUEENS* WHO SHOW UP FULLY FOR OURSELVES.

Haeley Mariah

BLESSINGS QUEEN

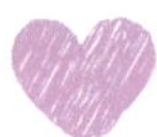

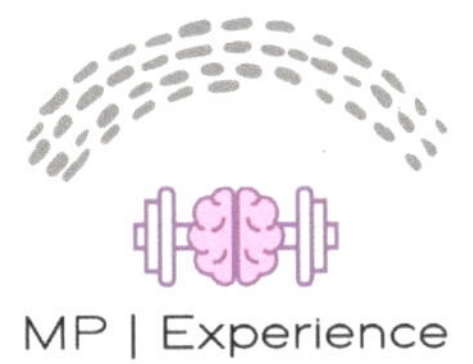

BELIEVING IS THE ANSWER. BECOMING IS THE SOLUTION. SELF-WILL IS THE GAME CHANGER.

Haeley Mariah

BLESSINGS QUEEN

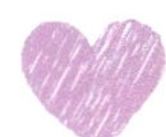

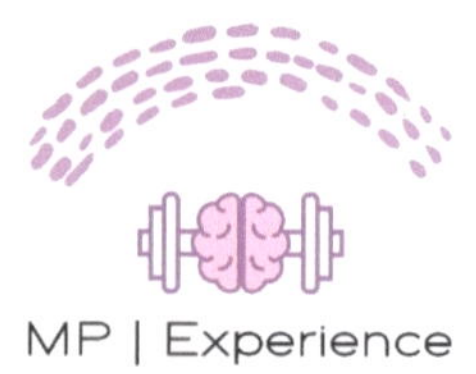

I AM... ENOUGH
I AM... LOVED
I AM... BEAUTIFUL
I AM... IMPORTANT
I AM... VALUED
I AM... GROWING
I AM... HEALING
I AM... A QUEEN

Repeat as many times as you need until you believe it.

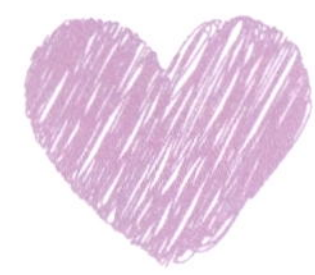

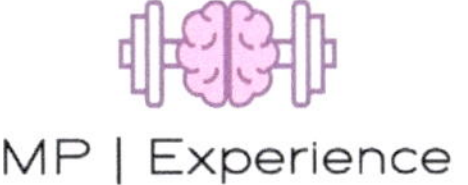